Andrey Bakuley

HOW I BECAME A VEGETARIAN

OR MY EASY 21 DAYS CHALLENGE

Cover and book design by Andrey Bakuley
Cover photo © Andrey Bakuley
Copyright © 2018, by A.Bakuley. All right reserved.
ISBN:9781980895053
Imprint: Independently published
74 pages

Disclaimer
This book is a given example of personal vegetarian experience. All facts, science conclusions or any other statements cannot be used by a person as a treatment or any part of remedy or other healthy solution. Before taking decision to be a vegetarian, you must see your physician or any other doctor related, in order to evaluate potential risk of being vegetarian.

This book does not discriminate any person according to any way of life, religion, outlook or other belief. The book is exceptionally a description of personal experience and does not guarantee any result expected after reading this book.

PREFACE

This is the book about unique personal journey....

An absolutely breathtaking experience, helping me to look back to my life and realize all the beauty of this transformation once again, share it with you, live it again and tumble to the mystery and absolute beauty of nature, to our Planet and fabulous life around.

It was one of the regular days to wake up and notice something different in me, something that I could not even predict. It was strange feeling for me that I wanted to become vegetarian.

This story is describing all my experience of my own way of changing to an animal lover from a regular meat lover.

I am glad to share with you my ideas, my thoughts, my feelings in all my transformation period. Here, I show you all possible tools for transformation like changing habits, meditations and meal planning.

If you still think about becoming vegetarian, but you do not know how or you have contradictions in the family or any other reason that may stop you from progressing like fears of lacking any substantial food elements, my experience may help you in this point. Some definite examples are given in this book to help you understand more about food and get rid of any fear of missing proteins or useful fats.

May my story be inspiring for you and with all hopes let it get you to a new challenge, a new unique journey leading you to an absolutely new way of life.

Table of Contents

The beginning.

This story begins from nowhere. I was a regular person with normal simple life wishes and habits, eating mostly everything, having some extra weight as it happens when someone is getting older, experiencing regular seasonal flu and other unpleasant things until a certain moment. From year to year, I never thought what was good and what was not.

I guess as many of us, I had a wrong feeling from time to time, and I knew that unlike anybody else, my body was different, my life was different and actually, I even didn't know what to do.

And real crisis came. Slowly and slowly, I was realizing that things were not going ok and I started to search myself by means of looking into myself. I can say, this search has no end, has no deadline, has no measurements, especially because it is a search of ourselves, an inside of ourselves, and an outside of ourselves, and it doesn't matter which one of those above, because the search is done by us and it is only about us.

I was coming from source to source with the will to understand the essence of things around me, why people were not happy or unhealthy or many other negative points they had in their life. By that time, I had already tried many things, listened to yoga lectures, but never tried myself, and I read specific literature and watched tons of movies. More and more questions, I had in my head.

After some time passed, I understood that I had to become a vegetarian. I did not realize what I really wanted, but I had to. Do you feel the difference? This "had to" came from the general trend circulating now in public, being so much advertised in social ways and speculated so many times all over internet and life. I definitely decided that I had to be a vegetarian. I had no clue what was this and how to cope with this, and what were the consequences of this diet, but I definitely decided that I had to.

I started. Several days, maybe even weeks I did not eat meat, but I ate eggs, fish and other seafood. Everything was under control, because I was thinking that everything was under control and I felt something new about me.

Meanwhile, I was developing my consciousness to a certain level, I was quaffing specific information from around and definitely I was trying to get more insights on what I had already known.

How it usually happens, I was invited to visit relatives and have dinner with them. It was time of holidays and there were lots of dinners coming one after another during this short period. One dinner after another and I was looking at the table as the tiger at the warm flesh. All those meatballs, sausages, fishes and everything were so beautifully decorated, even sparkling with stars on the table. I am not mentioning smell here, it was simply gorgeous.

Finally, I decided not to keep vegetarian diet, it was enough for me and I said to everybody that I was going to eat meat again at the next evening dinner when we gathered again and suddenly, I found lots of excitements and even appraisals for that from different people. I read in their eyes that "finally you came back and you are the one of us".

Usually, you may find someone's reaction to be very strange and you don't know exactly why they behave this way and what are their motivations for such positive or negative evaluations of your vegetarian way of life. But the most terrific thing here is that you don't know your motivation yourself and this is crucial point. Just imagine, you decided to become vegetarian or even vegan that is even more shocking, and suddenly, you realize that this is for nothing indeed, because you don't feel real motivation. How come are you going to get proteins or vitamins or some other minerals for your beautiful hair or nails? Sometimes, we don't know exactly how vitamins act and how the body digest minerals, but we are already afraid of losing something that we don't even know exactly how those things work. We think that we are getting minerals and everything, but we never know how. If we could know how, it would be clearer for us that everybody is different and just getting the vitamins in theory do not guarantee that we really are able to get them. This is related not only to meat or fish; actually it is related to the whole digestive system. If there is any misbalance in our body in digestive system, we are not going to receive any type of good minerals for ourselves just because they are not going to be properly digested. Anyway, we do not give up and still think about them and feeling fear of losing them.

Some big part of myths comes to our mind from our surrounding, our friends, communities, relatives; nobody and never was brought up as vegetarian and no one knows the way to be a vegetarian exactly. This is like driving the new road where we don't feel comfortable because we don't know the way itself, it is very new for us and we need to learn how to live with this. Definitely, we are getting beyond the comfort zone, since we decide to live this life and keep our way without surrender.

This is why, I am lovely sharing with you my way, my experience showing that many things are absolutely possible and without giving it a try you are not going to understand the new road. I am not going to teach you how to keep vegetarian way of life and you need to decide yourself the best things for you; I just want you to understand the essence of those things and the way how it works. The way how to build your balanced diet, its purposes - all that is not the aim of this book, because the aim of this book is to help you believe that this is possible and this is simple.

Going back to my attempts of eating meat again, I believed that this was so much difficult to stop eating meat, fish and eggs, all that was like an impossible mission at all. I was so much confused, because I had already smelt this scent of changes and felt myself new. You know this magic feeling, when you change yourself for better and you do some steps for development, and it exactly motivates you when you look at yourself and see the results. Here, I felt totally different. It was a feeling of frustration, missing motivation, just five minutes of eating and I was back to my old way of life again. Anyway saying honestly, the desire to feel flesh in my mouth was a way stronger than all my feelings about my motivation.

By that period of time, I had already understood that I could not find proper motivation for myself and I still did not understood why I needed to be vegetarian.

After a while, I started to feel difference comparing periods of eating and not eating meat. It happened suddenly after dinner, when I felt it very heavy in my stomach. I was amazed that I had never felt it before. It was so strong and uncomfortable heaviness and laziness, I felt like I lost comfort, it was definitely terrible feeling. My logic started to work in this direction, looking for reasons why that was so much powerful and crucial for me and deep inside of myself I realized that this was harming me and the energy of the flesh that I took was not so good and the reason why I never had felt it before was only because I had had nothing to compare before. Eating meat was a habit, and I never even thought about this difference.

Habit is a very interesting thing. From one side we know everything about habits, and we think that all is clear, but after a while I understood that I knew nothing about habits at all. This is very interesting, and

I am going to show you this in this book how it works in practice.

Finally, I got the conclusion that eating meat or any other creature was something harmful for the body, because I understood if veggie food made me feel easier and more comfortable, so then it must be very helpful and useful food. And on the contrary, meat food brought me to laziness and I felt uncomfortable. It means that this is something harmful. It was good that I understood all from that, but I did not know what to do with all that. It was ok for me to understand this harmless, but it was not ok for me not to be able to understand what to do with all that. So I was jumping among different theories, and I was trying to understand some methods, nothing worked for me for the only one reason - I did not understood my motivation, and this was something so personal and very deep inside. Instead of this, I was trying to understand things laying on the surface like trends, movements and different sayings about how it was disgusting to kill animals etc. and etc. Do we really know how meat comes to the supermarket? Some of you maybe found it out and had experience on how it happens but many of us do not think about this, which is normal in most cases. We come and see standard packing of flesh and we do not even feel what happened to this flesh before. So finally, those things about feelings "sorry" do not work for us as motivation, and I refer to myself, saying that it did not work for me as well. Now, let's imagine that we have so much empathy to creatures when it is well cooked or grilled, which is even stronger addiction when we eat grilled food due to the use of great amount of different species and herbs and whatever else to make it in the most delicious way. Usually, we don't eat meat as it is. Try to compare two types of cooked meat - the boiled one and the grilled one. There will be a big difference in taste. So, we completely forget here about pain and suffer of animals, because "grilled taste" can help forget everything, especially when we have no idea on what happened before. So, I didn't feel real motivation, for the same reason that I didn't have any real idea. I want to tell you that we should not blame ourselves for the lack of empathy. It is absolutely ok that we never think about this and there are many reasons behind like traditions, habits, behaviour or whatever else. We are all have a chance to change one day and we and only we may decide what to change, how to change and when to change.

Some time passed and things were still so simple for me. I smoked cigarettes, had alcohol and did not think that all those things were so much connected. One can chose life of being vegetarian and drink alcohol and smoke. This is what many people try and some of them are successful, and some not, it does not matter. The connection is not concluded in health options that alcohol and cigarettes can be harmful, this is something deeper and more fabulous to know and it comes to several thousands years ago practices of human experience.

Once, on a regular evening and before sleep I found "occasionally" a video on YouTube created by an interesting yoga community. This video was about yoga, about transcendental things and many other stuff, but since the movies were rather short, in about twelve minutes each, I got interested to see, and suddenly, I felt response inside of me, something sounded very much logical from what I heard, something was very known for me and I agreed with everything stated in that video and I would put my signature under every single word. For me it was like famous "wow" effect and I was very much impressed. I started to follow them and I listened to different and absolutely unknown things for myself, and karma effect was the easiest part from what I heard in those lectures and I was trying to understand what they were speaking about. When I was listening to them, I naturally paid attention to details and it was crystal clear fact for me in those details that all of them had absolutely different faces from what usually I used to see. I had the feeling that they had magically shining faces and the manner and the way to speak and to explain things - everything was so special. It made me believe them, I did not trust the words they said, I believed in results readable from their faces. Again, I used my logic and I was asking myself what those people did to be like that, so shining and so bright. The answer was simple; they did yoga and kept the lifestyle in a certain specific way unlike other people. They were all vegetarians; they watched what they did, what they thought and how they reacted to the environment in general. Even if bad things happened they knew how to react and what to do with those bad situations. This was the key answer for me. Everyday, I see people, different people of different manners, with different problems and attitudes, but I had a feeling that those ones were like aliens from different planet. This was for sure the real key for me.

I believed them so much that I started to think about stopping smoking and doing yoga and it was that much obvious for me, but realization of all those steps was almost impossible, and I did not really understood why. I was moving towards understanding my motivation much closer and I already knew that I needed yoga and I had to stop smoking definitely, but again and again the question "how to" was absolutely unclear for me. I was pushing myself, but it did not help me so much, I felt more upset after pushing myself. Anyway, the result was not clear. What was really clear in that situation that I did not want to stop in my progress and I worked harder and harder.

I was already trying meditations in my development cycle. I understood that yoga was something really far from me, but meditations as the part of yoga or even part of spiritual development were very exciting for me. I did many mistakes in mediation process, which was normal process in every study and did not matter what. I tried different techniques, used music, did it without music, did simple and more complicated postures. I had different feelings; I was thinking they were so much magic, but honestly to myself, I did not feel anything special and magic. It was focus and concentration, but nothing was special.

In one lecture on a different YouTube channel, I heard something what turned around my motivation and boosted so strong and actually became the idea for this book in the future. It was the explanation of why things did not work in meditations. Before I started to guess that meditation was very unique and sweet process, I did not know from which side to come to this magic box and open it. I wanted to feel it so much and I could not.

In general, we are all the bundle of habits behaving this or that way, and when we want to change ourselves, we want it immediately, not even thinking of things which have to be changed first. We want to have different life, or even small things - different and special meditation to chill us, but we are not ready to start doing things which we never did. Our deeds bring us to results and results are changing our view at ourselves. Without this movement we cannot change life, because we are not changing our habits as actions. If someone decides to stop eating meat for whatever reason, it is necessary to change habit and develop another habit of not to eat.

With small and small portions we are changing our habits and habits are changing our character and our new character is changing our life. This is why this famous saying comes with "if you want to change your life, start changing yourself from inside". Again, we come to the logic here about condition, if we change many of our habits, the bundle of habits, will it give us opportunity to change our life tremendously? The answer will be yes, because when someone is changing habits, it is impossible that life will be the same as life before this change started. This is an obvious dynamic process, and it helps us a lot to do many transformations with ourselves.

The question how to change habits comes. We understand that we are bundle of habits; we understand why we want to change it. When we change our habits, the motivation must be so strong and this is the rope which holds us over the surface in order to prevent us from falling down, because during our life experience we are forming our habits in so deep motivation, but it does not always mean that those habits are positive or healthy for us. Usually, it comes opposite. Most of habits we have, in our modern life are related to destroying our lives. We smoke, we drink alcohol, even some people take drugs, thinking of not heavy drugs are ok for them; some people do it with the strong belief that this is a really positive impact for them. For some moments, it may be positive, because smoking drugs may release some pain and it helps people to resist the pain and they still think that this is positive, but there is only small percentage of people who have prescriptions by the doctors based on some health issues, all the rest unfortunately not.

I would like to pay attention to one very important moment - there are no two same humans in the world existing, and if there is something good for the one, it does not mean that this is good for another one. How can we know that people smoking drugs are doing that kind of harm we are speaking here? It may be the only one way for someone to resist. It is too late for them to become clear in mind and do some healthy stuff. They simply have strong pain and they can't stand it. Of course, you will say, nothing is late and we need to perform as soon as possible some positive changes, but there are red lines when we cross them, it becomes too late. From another point of view, somehow we gain some power and a will to change ourselves even after red line is overstepped. In this case we definitely can agree that nothing is late and I really invoke you to believe in that. "Nothing is too late" idea is a powerful tool in our development, which gives us a good start and positive energy to begin any process of changes.

Eating no meat as a habit was formed somehow unconsciously in me, I just stopped eating meat without questioning myself. I continued meditation practices and listened to lectures of yoga teachers and monks and every time, I understood that I am on the right way of avoiding meat. That time I was still addicted to many things like fish or eggs, and I really believed in gaining proteins without even single knowledge of mechanism how it worked, how those amino acids developed proteins in us or how food was combined with other food, I just believed in that public sayings: "if you want muscles, you must take meat, if you want bones, you must take fish, if you need brain, you must take eggs and etc." Something did not work there and I felt myself still not good. Jogging in the morning, I felt sometimes not so healthy or very much exhausted, especially after warming up with some talks about how this was harmful for the body not to eat meat. For the body? Who are we? Only the body? This was what I was thinking, I am the only body and the rest of the world was separate substances from me, and here I were, and that was me as my body, my thoughts were like that until a certain moment, the moment of understanding meditations in a different way. I feel so good now remembering that moment of meditation, you know, guys, I am pausing writing this book now, because I want to go and meditate and feel this sweet moment again. See you in next chapter devoted to meditation.

Meditation.

There is no sense to explain you what the meditation is and how it is performed, and some of you may know it even better than me. There is plenty of different forms and types, postures and ways to perform, singing mantras, listening to chilling music or sounds of nature. All of this for sure brings a lot of positive vibes.

Since, I started to study it with one of my favourite teachers, and where I took online classes of meditation, I learned classics and it was very new for me, because I saw and I heard things for the first time in my life and they looked so strange for me. The first strange thing came from the posture. Before I was sure that there were postures with open hands directed up to the sky and suddenly, I heard that posture should be with my hands clasped in front of me down, my legs to be in a certain position where my foot was on the knee in a sitting position, and it was rather painful for the knees and joints. Anyway, I tried all of this and I was thinking at the moment of meditation how come this was possible to perform that strange posture and disconnect my mind off the world and concentrate. Everything was so strange.

Time past and it was definitely not so long and I got used to the posture, I would rather say that my body got used to the posture and I really started to feel that my mind was different from my body. It was strange feeling to have them separated. Before I was always sure that mind, body and personality were the same and there was no separation. This can be a good key to understanding how to open the first door of the aspect that I was saying before in the previous chapter about habits.

Let's come back to meditations, which is the one of the most beautiful and sacral processes in this beautiful world. After, I stopped feeling myself uncomfortable in that specific posture, I got absolutely new experience, I felt something strange inside. Every time, there were colorful splashes in front of me when breathing in and out, or some pleasant moments inside, and it was very hard to explain those feelings. I felt the feeling of "first love" without any reason. I was sure before that people needed to do some actions and to meet opposites to feel this love feeling again and again, and because of adrenaline and all those chemistry, but here it came so easily and unexpectedly. This was a beautiful feeling; it was without any reason, just the feeling without any reason. I knew nothing about mechanism of this feeling and the reasons of coming, but I was enjoying this beautiful feeling and for the first time in my life, I felt as a male that I can feel something very emotional in my heart. Usually, women are the first to feel that kind of emotions and any possible delicate emotions comparing to the men. So many times, I used to hear that I needed to develop, to open my heart and to listen to the things and the feelings with my open heart, not only with my mind, I never understood what those people meant that moment saying me that and how it was possible to feel with my heart. Try to stop and feel with your heart something. It may sound ridiculous, quite often we can't because we feel and identify things with our mind, we see objects, we evaluate them, we consider something and our mind gives us a certain conclusion afterwards. But here it goes without mind and evaluation, we don't think during meditation, we just meditate, and suddenly, we feel the "first love" and it is like we fall in love with the entire world. Every time we are connected to something powerful in our meditations. You may believe me, when you feel this for the first time in meditation, it will impress you so much that you will never forget it and you will want to come back to this more and more and it will be filling you from inside. You can do it in the morning, before going to work or study and you will be different. It is a charger. Do you remember your first feeling of love with somebody? How was it beautiful? We feel so much charged and we have power to do so many things, sometimes incredible things, we feel like dancing, we feel like jumping, it does not matter what else we feel like, it brings us a great amount of happiness from inside. This is exactly the feeling from the inside we gain every day after meditation. I think, this is what people claim to be "God is love", this is exactly love we feel to the God and entire World, we feel in love with everybody, until something poisons us and we forget this feeling until next meditation. In next meditation, we may not feel something special, because poisoning can be so strong and it can prevent all the flow of pure energy to us and we will not feel it, and it is normal, this is the process of development, and I think this is normal for all of us and we have all that so different, because we have different classes in our life to study, depending on our gains in the past.

Practically thinking, I understood, that all those beautiful feelings came to me as a pure divine energy; they gave me so much powerful energy to perform things in life. That's exactly the way how we feel energy and how we feel energy with different centers in our body. They are called chakras and since "heart" feelings are related to Anahata chakra, known also as a heart center, probably this center started to be cured in me. There is belief that when we feel with heart, we feel reality, and this is because we are able to feel it in more delicate way, and we can evaluate things more clear, deeper and easier. It could be very much possible, but the main idea was not to be so much discerning, the main idea was to feel this love to entire things around myself and now you will understand what I mean here.

I was progressing with this love feeling more and more until one day it gave me understanding that I and the surrounding world is absolutely the same. Definitely, I felt that I was of the same energy as other creatures surrounding me and this was the real motivation to become vegetarian, because we apparently feel really the same as other lives. I started to look at fish in a supermarket, for me it stopped to be just a food, because I looked in the eyes of so called fresh fish and I felt that it had been killed. It was suffering on its own way, suffered and felt pain. This was so amusing discovery for me! I looked at the eggs and I understood there were very much less energy, because it was small and probably not fertilized. I felt that I could not break the egg any more and destroy another creature anyway. I looked at mosquitos or fly, for me they stopped being just annoying insects, they were even like friends doing their own tasks and things in their lives. I looked at the ants penetrating into my kitchen as troops and I understood them that they had their own consciousness and this consciousness made them do the things which we consider as disgusting because they are usually dirty etc.

But excuse me! This is their own level of consciousness and they come this way because they have to come. Try to put your finger in front of them and kill some of them and you will see how they change roads and directions. Why? This is because their consciousness is pretty enough to understand that they have to live and they want to survive. If they have the will to live, who has the right to stop their life? It can be the one who is not conscious enough to understand and feel that this creature wants to live. Unfortunately, usually among people it is normal practice to kill and it is not ok, but it is clear. Many of us were not brought up and were not enlightened with this feeling of union with other creatures. God and nature give us hints sometimes as suffering, diseases, but we are still far away from this understanding, ignoring them, because we don't even think about that this is for real.

When we suffer because of killed creatures, it is not some punishment from God, it is important to understand that there is absolutely different perspective. We, as humans are the same creatures as well and it is not punishment, it is dissonance with our potential in our development. When we come to this Earth as humans we have more potential to open our hearts and be enough conscious not to kill other creatures. The ant has one task in its life, very simple, we, humans have different tasks - we need to create and not destroy. So, when we go away from our main goals as humans and we don't use our potential from the Divine to create and make this world beautiful we suffer due to ourselves in different forms and we have some psychological or physical disorders.

I was thinking about some statements, and I heard before that we are humans have canine teeth inside and we have them for the reason that we have to eat meat, but this comparison is the same as if we would consider our tail in our vertebra or nails as claws remaining as the reasons to eat flesh because we have something common with animals. It does not mean that we need to come back to our past experience when we needed to survive using any type of our instruments as canine tooth to eat some flesh to survive. Today, we have already been changed and our civilization moved forward enough to understand that we don't need those things anymore with us and finally any meat can be substituted for the sake of preserving another life. We have become pretty smart about life and we definitely know that we have enough variety in our life to use necessary elements for ourselves without taking another life.

You will see very big benefit for being so smart and refusal from meat. Nature will start to bloom in you with all positive vibes and it will give you all potential to survive without suffering.

Energy.

There is another aspect in having flesh to be eaten, and this is the energy or the information provided to your body from different creatures. There is good saying: "we are what we eat". Somehow it is really true. We are gaining information from another form of life into us together with cells. Same way we are getting information even from the vegetarian food, it depends how grass was planted and grown and how many chemicals were used to plant those seeds. Everything what we eat, we let this information create us. With meat this is even more serious, because we take the energy of killing and information of last moment of this creature as fear or pain will be transferred to us. After we start feeling some fear or anger transformed into different lighter forms of course, but still we are gaining and gaining it and it brings even more depression. This is the way the nature speaks to us that we have to stop eating other conscious lives.

Speaking about energies, I would like to raise some more things and share them with you. They are taken from the Vedic culture and they explain many things in a bit different perspective.

They are simply called as energies of nature or "Prakriti" (परकृति) in Sanskrit language. Their mechanism is rather complicated to understand, but I will try to explain them in a simple way. They are divided into three ways (Guna): "Sattva" or light sacral and pure energy with love which is a prototype of our thin energy form of living as our positive emotions and pure love to entire surroundings. In the middle of this range we have "Rajas" which is energy of dynamism and movements. I am not an expert in those traditional Vedic things, but as much as I understand this energy creates movements in us and may direct it into positive and negative aspect. This is like crossing the roads where you may chose, but this choice as a tool will be regarded as a movement. The third energy is "Tamas" and this is black energy and it is considered to destroy. This is paradox here caused by misunderstanding of things, because "Tamas" is not something bad and life needs it for the reason of creation and destroy cycle. Question here what do we chose, because food being as "Tamas" energy can lead us to destroy much faster than "Satva" food. At the same time "Tamas" black energy is a very powerful aspect, being a rough energy which may lead to a rather solid habit creation. "Tamas" food is coming from meat, fish and eggs, other creatures are included here as seafood, also alcohol and cigarettes, everything what brings human to satisfaction through destroying. Some other food may be considered as "Tamas", but I will not go so deep and if you are interested you may surf internet today and find profound information.

There is no doubt that it is harmful to our body. Same as our body, it is harmful to our soul as well. Official science doesn't know it exactly, and we consider that all science in this case is us and we only may feel the difference of "before" and "after" based on our own experience. It is possible to make conclusion only in comparison. It does not mean that we may feel that once, it does not mean that we may feel it at all. Again, we are all different. It is so much possible as well, that we will not feel that for the reason that we need this experience and we need to eat meat and other "Tamas" food, because this is the essence of the life conditions today. It is rather hard to survive somewhere in the North Pole and to be vegetarian, just for very simple reason - there is no such a variety of green, orange, red and whatever food and those northern people they have to eat meat to survive. Some people need to do it for some healthy reasons and they don't have time or chance to change and for them this is the only option.

This is why when we become vegetarians; we have no right to judge people who eat meat in front of you. It is a multilevel factor of becoming vegetarian as you see from this book that we need to be patient. When we eliminate meat from our body, we become more patient and empathic to other people, we start understanding them deeper and differently, we understand how it is difficult to start new habit destroying the old one which is rather firm and sustainable.

From my side I should admit that it does not mean that the motivation will come from the meditation. I am pretty sure that some people may have this empathy to creatures without meditations, but for the most of us having already been so deep in "Tamas" energy for a rather long time and having loaded ourselves with some other black energies during our life, we need to be very deep inside and we really need to work to avoid black energy as much as possible.

Besides alcohol and cigarettes, meat, fish and eggs, there are some surprising things for us as onion and garlic. They are considered to be "Tamas" food and even very strong "Tamas" food. As I said before, it is rather complicated to understand energies just in one chapter, and the aim of the book is a bit different, but this is important to know and in next book I will explain more about energies based on my experience in order to reveal this separately and detailed for those ones who might be interested much more, especially taking into consideration that "Tamas" or "Rajas" are not only about the food, this is our way of thinking, our positive or negative attitude.

So, why it is so important to understand energies and mechanisms of their activity? This is because, since we live in those three energies (Guna) all the time, we need to use them as a tool helping us more and more, especially if we want to go away from eating the meat. We stop eating "Tamas" food and we understand that we are less and less connected to this energy. Instead, we are gaining energy of "Sattva" eating fruits and vegetables, corns and cereals and many other things.

It does not mean that some of those energies are bad or good, it should not be considered this way. The idea is to accept the fact that all energies are needed at a certain level. First of all, we have to understand the contrast between them. Second, this is the normal life cycle. Tamas will serve human body, and actually not only human after death in order to start decay process and bring the body to initial form and mix it with the Mother Earth. When we stop eating "Tamas" food and then when we come back to eating it again, we feel the difference. It can be manifested as feeling of heaviness in digestion system, laziness, a strong desire to sleep. Why? As I explained in previous sentence aim of "Tamas" is to destroy and bring creature to initial form, to decompose into atoms or even less.

Let's do a logical conclusion from the above mentioned statements. If we load ourselves with "Tamas" food, we boost our decay process and we do get older much faster just because this is the essence of "Tamas", we feel this destroy, we feel this black energy and this energy accelerates the destroying process in our body much faster.

There are many contradictions about this and some people claim something like: "Look at the animals, predators, tigers, lions, sharks and many others. They eat all this and "Tamas" energy does not destroy them, they are strong and fast. They are ideal in their creations".

My respond to those statements is rather simple. Yes, they do and yes they are, but, first let's not forget that animals live in full compliance with nature, they do not feed their kids with chips or soft drinks, they do not sit many hours in front of the screen, they live in nature and nature gives them tools to survive and they are in the middle of this life cycle, even if one has to eat another one. We cannot compare ourselves to animals, we are not animals, we think different and our consciousness is different. We do not have those strong claws and fangs. Nature gave us absolutely other tools as pure mind and ability to see things more clearly and the main tool given to us from nature is ability to feel love, which is a starting point of all consideration of the environment. We are here to be more above of those natural processes like simply to eat and eat everything. We are here not only to eat. If someone wants to compare human with animal because lions are getting proteins from meat or something like that, it will be honest to compare lions to humans in full aspect. Do lions do so many things in their lives like humans? Do they have targets and ambitions like humans? Do they have this ability to love their kids until the end of the life like humans? The list can be extended, and to make it short, the idea is to show that we are not lions or other predators and we have wider opportunities and abilities in our lives. Our consciousness is much higher comparing to any of the animals. There are some animals with consciousness like elephants, dolphins, cows, some types of birds. They are not predators and they have different diet for the reason that nature created them in different manner and they are already one step above predators and on the way to human.

There is one more interesting fact, whether or not you believe in reincarnation. It is clear that our soul is elevating all the time and progressing from simple forms, from some creatures to humans and even more. Again, this is another topic for discussion, but definitely we feel this line in the fact that predators are staying on their certain level of progress and after being predators they should do great breakthrough and start moving to humans, which is not easy for them. So, finally we understand and we should leave an animals example apart, we are simply not animals, we can feel, we can sing and play music, even more, some of us can create music or paints, we create the World, we are able to change the World. We have big power, very big power; we have such a great power to create the same way as to destroy. Think about this, please, you all have power. Think please, what you would do with this power.

All this was in my mind while doing meditations one after another and feeling more and more that I did not see any difference between me and a tree or a bird or just another person. I understood more and more about Prakriti as main energies of Nature, and this is because we are all created out of the same energy.

There is another bigger aspect in respect of energies. When I felt that I was the same as the entire world, I started to see things not only as a physical aspect, but also as energy. When I looked at the laptop or lamp near me, I understood and felt more that this was not only piece of physical substance like metal, plastic or glass. I started to see it consisted of parts and atoms and all that was just a physical aspect of the energy from the environment. Looks complicated? Absolutely not. Do you remember how Prakriti works? Energy is taken and under certain circumstances they are transformed into some natural, organic and inorganic materials. You know that glass was created of sand with fire. But what is sand? Sand was a mineral created by nature and fire is plasma containing huge amount of powerful energy. Just think! Fire is a substance with the ability to heat to several thousands degrees. Both components are created and taken from nature and finally we have this magical transformation into a glass. Later, humanity found the way to create glass out of other materials and they became to be a glass, but if we look deeply and more attentively to a glass, we will understand this is still sand transformed with fire. Now imagine that sand as a piece of mineral has atomic nature and there is movement, always a movement, and it is called vibrations and any movement creates energy. We know it from the lessons of physics. The conclusion here is that it contains initial energy provided by nature. Before sand became sand it had been in different forms and by means of a certain power of nature it had been transformed to sand. Same way it was with energy. It was in huge mineral having some part of energy of the Universe and, suddenly, it was transformed to sand keeping the same energy, then sand was transformed to a glass. It means that same energy spilled over to a glass. Now we can agree that absolutely anything what we can touch and even what we cannot touch contains same energy.

Logical question comes here, and if all is the same energy, travelling from one form to another one, why physical aspects are transforming into different forms, and why energy repeating the physical aspect is spilled over into another physical aspect being transformed and this physical aspect is different, but energy is the same. In other words, why sand was transformed into glass, but energy remains the same. We just do not see that energy transforms as well and it is being transformed as sand by means of fire. This is why natural energy is subdivided into three aspects (Gunas) as "Sattva", "Rajas" and "Tamas". This is why they exist in order to change the world and transform it into different forms.

Now it is clearer that food is the same energy and other creations are of the same energies and when creatures are killed, it means immediate transformation in the body and energy. The creature was eating grass and feeling happy and next hour it felt strong pain and, finally it was killed. Energy of happiness transformed into energy of destroying and pain. This energy remains in the flesh and it is coming from place to place until it gets to the shelves of supermarkets.

Now we understand more that being a vegetarian is not only a modern trend, it does not mean something like to avoid a diary food, because it is animal production. Nothing is bad with milk; there is no pain in milk production. Of course, I do not mean a big plant dairy production, where cows are heavily used and may feel pain. I mean the case, when we interact with the cows in the normal and natural way and they give us milk with love and dedication. There is no energy of destroy and it may really happen that a cow may love you and give you a good energy with the food it produces, in this case, it is a milk. But, if we load ourselves with the energy of destroy and sorrow, sooner or later we will feel it and get it, when the scale of energy proportions in us will prevail to be more negative than positive. Energy is the king in this aspect and I hope more or less you understand how energy works and what kind of influence it brings.

We are touching the aspect of the energy in this book specifically for food explanations, but I am sure that it will logically end up with many other aspects and it can bring you to understanding that it is not only food being important in terms of understanding the energy, but also other things surrounding us, especially personal things may contain and they do contain energy which can be either positive or negative for us depending on what we did in the past.

We described the aspects of energies in things surrounding us and there is one more important energy for us which is inside of us, we are the energy by itself the same way as we are the creatures of the same Universe that created us. We are the energy transformed into a certain rough form same as sand being transformed into a glass, as you remember from the previous example. We have bodies, they are all different from the beginning, given to us by our parents, because we have been attracted to the same energy of our parents and our parents attracted us in the manner of their present energy. So what does it mean? It means that children are coming to the parents in different moments of their life and they can be different accordingly to the energy of their parents. When parents smoke, drink alcohol and do many other "Tamas" things, then they attract the kids to bring the same properties to reflect and return the same to their parents in double, when parents need those lessons. And the same way, when parents live "Sattva" life or they try to change to it, which is not easy for people, they will attract children with the same characteristics to life. Why am I explaining all this here? I do this for the reason that we need to understand that all of us come with different energies, depending on our relatives and ourselves and the reason why you are reading this book now might be because your parents all the time have been strong meat eaters and you came to their life to help them change themselves and you have your energy inside of you with this initial point to start the process of transformation for your relatives and to stop eating meat in order to save other creatures and you will do it to be followed as a good example. It is true, if you want to change and your relatives do not want to or have not changed yet. So we can conclude, that we all coming to life with different starting point and with different energies as a part of Universe and this is a diversity. Maybe you started reading this book, because you had been the meat eater in the past life or even in present life or there can be even stronger fact that you had been the hunter and now you need to correct this. Our soul, our spirit always helps us with this. It gives us the key, where to go and how to go to a new challenge and, finally how to change our life, our present life.

Suddenly, we stop eating meat, other creatures like fish and eggs and we understand by means of some unique internal feeling that we change and our energy changes and we start feeling transformation. I personally think that it happens for two reasons, which are combined into one reason at the end. The first one is that we stop loading ourselves with the energy of killing and suffering and the second one is that we transform our personal energy inside of us for the reason of feeling compassion to other creatures. The less we load ourselves with so-called "black energy", the more we move our energy from the black side to the light one.

I was sceptical for the first period of time when I was told by my teachers that my energy supposed to be changed, and even then I did not feel how I lost this moment of transformation inside of me. I had been already transformed and I still did not believe in that so strong change and it made a big influence on me and people surrounding me. I woke up with the understanding that there were people around asking me advice how to eat without meat, how to become vegetarians or vegans.

In order to have more idea about how some of those energies work in you it is needed to go deeper to the science of yoga or any other valuable spiritual sciences, and believe me, you will find a lot of interesting stuff there for yourselves in order to understand the question. We are touching this only slightly and we are creating the idea of how all those things work. From my side, I can add the fact that energies interact not only in food combinations; they are connected also to many other aspects, like behavior and our psychological state. All of this is interrelated and make influence on each other, but definitely it is clear that food plays significant role in our own transformation. After the food is "clean" from black energy, it is much easier to practice many things as yoga or meditation or just pray or whatever else, and all those things come much faster and easier and change our consciousness. From the other hand, meditation or yoga may bring people to vegan life, because they clean the black energy from inside and one day you may wake up with the full understanding that you are vegetarian not because of a trend and people who are in social networks promoting healthy way of life, even though it is also a good reason, but there will be also another feeling, it will be a feeling of compassion to alive creatures, and you will see that you cannot eat them anymore.

Following habits.

One day I started to guess that there are certain rules in our body helping us create our habits, so I decided to do an experiment and see how it really works.

Many times I heard about twenty one days rule helping us change any possible habit and create something new instead. When I did it with meat, I did not think so much, but this thing became my internal engine, making a sort of understanding inside of me that there was something definitely mystical, and somehow it should work. So, I started creating blogs on Instagram, and it was an amazing beginning for my experience. I had no clue how to blog on Instagram, how to attract people, and why it should be interesting for them, but suddenly, I realized for myself that it became very helpful. It was some sort of psychological aspect, when I started my blog and people read me, and I could not break rules and change my way, at least I had to finish those twenty one days and see the result and many people were expecting the same.

My first experience I started with jogging and I did between seven to ten kilometers, which was around four and a half to six miles of regular run. I did it every day and I took pictures of surroundings, being amazed with the natural beauty I made comments and shared my feelings, and my whole experience with other followers.

One Saturday morning, I woke up at seven and at around eight I was tying my snickers' laces preparing a plan in my head. I decided to do a kind of challenge and see how my body had changed for the time of global transformation and how my twenty one days jogging affected me. I started with my all electronic helpers, distance and calories counters, headphones and an amazing music inside. I planned a route and it was like a dancing and not even jogging, I found myself feeling exhausted when I exceeded eight kilometers, which were around five miles and I decided to continue after some short drinks of pure water. I clearly remember when I said to myself that it was not my limit and I had to go more. Many of you may know this feeling called as a "second breath", so this was exactly the case, and I was running under the sun and high temperature. I finished twelve and a half kilometers, so it was seven and a half miles, first time in my life such a pure run. I stopped and felt immediately that I could do more, but I pulled myself away from this idea, because I clearly realized that there was a limit and it might end not so well for me. Those long distance run was a good and clear proof of some deep changes in my body, and I had never run so long in my life almost without stop and I had never felt so strong before. It was a very good feeling.

I started to do other probes with other twenty one days challenges and I found that they worked and changed people. They really form our habits and change to that ones what we want to be. Once you want to find yourself drinking a lot of pure water everyday, so just do it every day, follow your idea and approximately after eleventh day you will feel like you want to continue specifically this way and there is no other way for you and you really want it. After twenty one days you will not even think that you have been practicing a habit, it will be absolutely natural process for you, you will feel like you have been drinking water this way for all your life. This is an exact habit you want. So as you guess, you may form like this any habit you want. It is really extremely powerful instruments helping us construct ourselves from inside and outside the way we want. I really like the saying: "When we change our habits, changed habits change our character and our character changes our life". This is so true, and it makes us feel so strong and really believe in ourselves. Just imagine that you want to have something and before you have been dependent on somebody's help or any other circumstances and you have never known that this beautiful power is located just inside of you. We are human creatures who got used to imposing responsibility to somebody or something in case of failures, and we often bear responsibility when we have luck and something works for us and we say that this is because of us. In most other cases we may say that this is a nature or parents honor, or other relatives, friends, street, government, country whatever else, and we don't have even a single idea what is inside of us and how powerful we are from inside. The twenty one days changing instrument is just the only peak of the mount we may see, because quite often we don't need anything from outside to bring our ambitions to reality. I want this idea to be very clear with you guys, you should not think that in order to do something, you obviously need something special. The thing is that you don't need a new smartphone for a creation of a new thing in your life. It will not bring you anything besides the new device which you will forget in two or three months and you will be on the same stage as before. And on the contrary, try to survive with the thing you have, let it be the old one and let it be not so trendy and cool, but do the new target for yourself and finish this target and you will feel two things for yourself: a new gift and a strong power inside of you, which will let you complete your task with bare hands. Immediately you start feeling that in order to complete your challenge, you do not need new clothing, new snickers to do 6 miles of run or new smartphones to follow your calories. No, it will be different, you will feel very clearly that your level is high and everything came out from inside of you, you like the magician creating things from nothing. Many of us, and me in the past, spent a lot of money to lose weight and we come from one to another professional to have some magic advices and we have never asked ourselves, and suddenly, we just understand that we stop eating white bread and related products, drinking soda drinks and other sugar enriched drinks, we do jogging or other sports activity and this can be so much enough to lose couple of pounds for two weeks or something. Instead of buying and buying something, we stop buying, we don't buy special magic new trainer or pills to reduce fat, and we just don't buy "usual" things for us. Just think about how beneficial it can be for you, if you just stop buying, and instead of sweet drinks you start drinking water. At least you save money on pills, you save them on sweet drinks and you will be getting closer to your amazing clean and sound body. There is no smartphone, cosmetics, game, book or cool movie being able to compete to your sound and healthy body, and on the contrary to books, movies, games, cosmetics or smartphones, you need almost nothing to have your dream sound body. With the things surrounding us, we need to spend a lot and work a lot and be a bit in a positive meaning slavery. After doing experiments on different aspects, this idea became so clear for me that I almost need nothing, if I want to get this or that with my body. First you change your habit, character and then life. There is another cool saying I like: "If you want to have something you've never had in your life, start doing something you've never done in your life." This is very clear that change of habit makes us do something absolutely new and this may lead us to totally new results.

You know, I am not an expert in this field and I do not claim myself to be so, I just share my experience and I can agree that there are habits in our lives apparently much stronger than we can imagine, and it is really hard to resist them. They can be drugs or alcohol, they act on different levels of our chemical system and they create habits differently involving our feelings and emotions, our brain and our whole nervous system. So, in some cases, twenty one days may not be considered to be enough to easily change a habit. In most cases, we need an external help to do so, but from another side it depends on every separate specific case. First of all, we need to understand that probably we need some external help; it may be hard and in some cases even dangerous for life just to stop it. Second, we have to be stronger than others and be more than twenty one days patient and expect the result even after sixty or ninety days. Be stronger than others and express a will. What I love about cats and same about big cats, the fact that they are extremely patient. For me patience is some sort of wisdom. Unfortunately, they are not vegetarians, and they have to be extremely patient to strategically capture their next victim sacrificed for another life survival, but they are not humans and they are far away from the possibilities of human in creating unique lives and preserving other lives. However, there is something we may learn from them, and this something is patience. They need this to survive; we need this to variate our possibilities and use them in some specific cases of our life.

I used Instagram blogging to have my habits controlled and followed, and strictly complete them and share results. I tried food, I was running, and studying languages, since I had a lot of people addicted to travelling and many other things and in most cases I saw that twenty one days rule really worked. One of the last changes of habit was related to avoiding gluten food in vegetarian lifestyle and exclude so many food from my schedule was really hard. I remember how I felt before eleven days and I was ready to eat stone and wood, because I wanted those gluten pasta, pizza and whatever else more and more and after eleven days, I felt clearly that my body and my cells did not require this type of food anymore, so something like salad, a raw salad spiced with some pepper or oil was absolutely enough for me. This is how it works and it was absolutely clear for me.

So, if we want to change not only to be a vegetarian, but we want to accustom ourselves to something else like reading books every day for 20 minutes or drinking two glasses of pure water in the morning before meal and not during the meal, you will benefit a lot.

When we change our habit, we need to understand why we do it. Our motivation should be strong enough, and besides motivation we need to answer the question "how to?". Since we decided to become a vegetarian, we need to figure out how we are going to substitute elements which we used to get from the regular meat food.

Food combination.

This chapter is very important for understanding and I will try to be as clearer as possible to explain why it is so important. It is going to be about elements in food and substantial meals for vegetarians.

At first time, I was a bit frustrated with the idea of avoiding specific food and missing elements in it as a result. Somehow, I was thinking that food and meals would be boring and it really happens like this, because just imagine, you have the same regular meal seven days a week with some definite food preparations and suddenly, missing half of regular meals. What do I have left? All those carbos and some fats, but almost no proteins and soon I might be under the risk of gaining extra weight, and this is what happened to me, because I felt boring somehow at the beginning and somehow, I decided that if I do not eat creatures, I will eat sweets, I will eat chocolate and more of something like that. It was a big mistake! No way! I gained extra pounds for just several months, much more than I had before.

So, before you switch to be a vegetarian, which is an amazing benefit for your life and body, I really recommend you to plan your food, really to plan it, to think how you would avoid this boring porridge or just regular boiled potato.

I love the saying of La Rochefoucauld: "To eat is a necessity, but to eat intelligently is an art" This is exactly what I mean here! You must create your food as a piece of art, it should be interesting for you and you should feel satisfied eating this food. You may agree with me that there is a big difference in having meal at some sophisticated restaurant, food served on the trendy plate or opposite way and just in the street, where it is rolled in a piece of paper. Same is with having meals at home or at work, anyway dishes should be served with love, where preparation should be a piece of art, so you could have a wish to grab your smartphone and do the picture for another social media post.

Beside all those esthetics, there is something else important to consider in this chapter. It is food itself and a combination of this food. Like this we need to know how food elements interact with each other, what is beneficial for our digestion and when we are going to have elements being digested and why.

An interesting story happens here. First you realize that there is much more variety in food that has to be applied, you meet absolutely new types of food, some of them you have never heard of before or at least have never considered them seriously. This was with me, I heard about many things, but always considered them to be beautiful fantastic stories unless I tried them all myself. This is how a lot of exotic stuff comes to your life and you never know how it may help you.

I am going to share some more tips with you and I think it is extremely important to keep the track of those things.

This is not a big secret that our bodies utilize proteins, fats and carbs and there are a lot of studies that proving different ways of combination and consumption. I am not going to go deep to that, since you may find today plenty of theoretic information, but practical significance of those food types is more important.

Proteins.

We all know that protein is a necessary element required by our body and it brings lots of constructive ways to build our body. We all need muscles, bones, regenerating cells and whatever else official science may prove. This is true, that we take a lot of proteins from flesh or eggs. Besides that, we also gain proteins from vegetables, fruits and greens, and we divide proteins into animal and veggies ones. In order to receive the necessary proteins we need a range of amino acids and this range depends on the purpose of what we grow: muscles, hair, nails and so on. Amino acids are so important and they play a significant role in the way of constructing proteins, it is similar to a specific code guiding our body the way the cells to be constructed. So, those acids are taking an important part in the general process of metabolism and there are types of acids that may be produced by our bodies and some of them, called essential amino acids are not produced by our body and we need to take them from our food. This is so crucial and so sensitive idea and we need to remember that missing even one type of amino acid may mislead our body protein formation and harm our body in the future very easily. This is why we need to be very clear and confident that we get enough of sufficient food with all the necessary essential amino acids. The list of those amino acids is not that long and quite easy to keep track of them. They are valine, tryptophan, isoleucine, arginine, leucine, histidine, lysine, methionine, phenylalanine and threonine. We need all of them in full and necessary dose. Before we reveal the way how we are going to get them, we have to take into consideration the fact that our body needs to be able to receive the acids in proper way and in full amount. I mean here that we have to watch antagonistic food that may also lead to destructive process of certain elements in our metabolism. For example, there is a belief that coffee may ruin calcium in our body rather easily and this is why it is often recommended to get some mineral water during coffee sessions. In some countries like Italy it is an absolute rule to have mineral water when you visit restaurant or even a small coffee shop. Same effect may come up with acids, which are more difficult to be destroyed, but from another side, it is also quite difficult to synthesize them from food, if it is not taken properly. This is why we need to watch how we eat and what we eat, and besides the fact that it is quite difficult to remember everything, there are still some simple recommendations that may be used as simple helpers: smoking and alcohol. It is enough to stop those two habits and you will be guaranteed to consume amino acids in the right way.

If you read this book, it means that you are interested for any possible reason to be vegetarian and amino acids taken from any type of creature are not the part of this book.

I would like to make a small notice also about difference between animal and veggies food in general.

It is size of portion. What I saw from other people and this is what happened to me as well that we even intuitively increase portions because we feel like our food is not so substantial and we have to eat a little bigger portion. Nothing happens when you eat big bowl of salad and then increase volume of beans, and all that looks extremely healthy and good, but it is quite easy to lose control over your consumption volumes and get deeper to the illusion that you do quite perfect. From the other side you start gaining for example a lot of belly fat not because of fat, saturated or trans fats, even though they also play some necessary role, but not so significant in this meaning, the much bigger effect comes from calories and calories are coming from portion size. Whatever theories you can see about good and bad cholesterol, fast and slow calories, if you seriously increase your calories intake, there will be no big difference for our bodies, because exaggerated consumption of calories will signal to our body to store calories for the hungry future. This is our evolution gift and almost whole humanity is like that, we store everything, if we do not use it properly. So the rule is very simple to remember:

If we want to lose weight, we have to reduce consumption of calories and it does not matter how, we just eat less

If we want to gain more weight (what happens as well) we increase the consumption of calories

If we want to control and keep the same weight for a certain period, we have to watch our calories not to decrease and not to increase them

So, depending on our wishes, we can choose. It also depends on the type of metabolism. We have to remember that we also spend calories alongside with their consumption and if you are extremely physically active, you may lose them quite fast and be confident that everything is under control. The metabolism peculiarities in a certain body may also specify the consumption portion of calories. A classic example, if some person has a big mass of muscles, the consumption of calories will be definitely bigger since the massive core needs more elements to supports muscle tissue and dynamic process in them, and on the contrary, if the person does not eat sufficient amount of calories, it may lead to disruption of muscle tissue, so called catabolism, which will destroy the muscles and person will become slim, and after that when he or she comes back to increased consumption of calories it may easily lead to fat and not to muscles, since it is quite difficult to gain muscle type tissue comparing to fat. This is what quite often happens to people, when they keep specific diet to reduce fat by means of decreasing calories, but doing so without a plan what quite often brings people back to fats with even more weight gain. I really recommend you to think about this and do some types of food plan in order to be sure that everything you do goes in a right way. To finish ideas about portion sizes we should logically understand that there is a difference in portions when we take proteins from veg food comparing to proteins from the animals, for example a hundred grams of lentils will bring you 9 grams (0.31oz) of proteins, comparing to chicken breast which may give around 25 grams (0.88oz) per same one hundred grams or three and a half ounces. It means that we have to take around 300 grams (10.5oz) of lentils to have similar amount of proteins to reach the similar amount as of chicken. A hundred grams (three and a half ounces) of chicken breast gives us 165 calories and the same hundred grams of lentils gives us 116 calories. It is quite easy to understand that in order to get the portion of 25 grams (0.88oz) of proteins we need to get 116 calories multiple to three, which is 348 calories and this is almost twice more than from chicken.

Finally, what we get:

100 grams (3.52oz) of chicken gives us 25 grams (0.88oz) of protein and 165 calories

300 grams (10.5oz) of lentils gives us 27 grams (0.95oz) of protein and 348 calories. Chicken is a winner here!

If we continue consumption of calories in the same manner, we will get a lot of weight practically very fast. It means that we have to take it under control and keep tracking of what we eat. And again, we look back to the saying of La Rochefoucauld about the art of eating. We need to be more creative and more intelligent. Personally, I think it is much more interesting to be more creative comparing to eating rudderless, it is more exciting to get knowledge on usefulness of things and constantly to get rid of dangerous stuff. The motivation here is very clear - we save Planet, we save animals and we eat more Eco style. One day we start to have Eco life. I don't know, if you believe in karma and other things related to that, but for me it is quite clear that I'd better use my brain and save lives comparing to eating things and be not so conscious about that. If I have fear that my meal is not so sufficient, I will study and will never come back to the idea of eating creatures again. For sure, there is plenty of benefits to be vegetarian.

Let's see practically how we can get proteins from veg food without such a big impact of calories on us. This is quite simple since we have to do two basic things:

Consider exactly what we eat

Be physically active.

Physical activity can be absolutely different among what you like, but it must be certainly regular in your routine. Yoga, gym, jogging, swimming or anything else can be very good, because 40 minutes of jogging will use about 500 calories from our body, and if we eat 300 grams (10.5oz) of lentils to get 25 grams (0.88oz) of proteins and 348 calories, we will burn those extra two portions of food in about 40 minutes of morning run, which is not too big in general. It depends on the way you run and weight and many other factors, but the average can be around those numbers. I recommend you to take a program of 21 days and run everyday and you will see that this is not just a theory; it really works, because consumption of calories is real, same as gaining. We are all different and it does not mean that all those advises will work for all of us, but much more important thing here is an explanation of the idea of things that sometimes we never think of.

There is another benefit from eating healthy. Just imagine that you stop eating junk food and start watching your meals and this benefit is related to your future very closely, because you teach your body to create different way metabolism, stomach is getting to a different way of food processing and it means that the more healthy you eat, the more metabolism quality you may have. When we speak about vitamins and minerals, we expect to get them from food, but when our body is full of fat it means that all our digestive system is dirty and unable to process and transform all food to essential minerals and vitamins. We fool ourselves quite often thinking that having an orange together with saturated fats will give us more vitamin C or A. Some of them yes, some no, it depends on many factors because the level of body pollution is different, habits are different. Someone smokes another one drinks alcohol and so on. We know from many sayings that "we are the one what we eat", and practically you can imagine that cucumber or carrot eaten on breakfast is converting literally to your cells and more over it helps to build our body with the same amino acids, proteins and minerals. A certain cucumber will become a part of our cells at the end. All the rest, mostly it is tissue after being squeezed is going to be out. So, this way we use all the advantage from food and the rest is going out. It is interesting to imagine, looking at carrot, which has different shape, form, it grows in different conditions and suddenly we do a bite and chewing it piece by piece and squeezing juice with fiber and now, please, just stop and think, use your internal microscope and understand that this juice consists of water and minerals and vitamins, acids and proteins and they are there, really there. They are different from eating cookies enriched with carotene from carrots, because it is hard to imagine how carotene can survive in the cookies processed in the oven with the temperature of 220 C degrees. We have so many things around that our imagination does not see in certain way and we are rather often confusing carrot and cookies and we think that they are both useful. They are, but they cannot be compared. It is simply impossible, we cannot consider carrot and cookies to the same level of usefulness, and I don't say that cookies are not useful; I say that we may be confused with different things. If we expect carotene from cookies same way as from the fresh carrot, there can be a doubt that they are really the same. There are technologies doing magic and keeping stuff to be fresh and s, substantial, but we are not always sure. In case with fresh carrot or other vegetables we are more ensured in getting real thing, almost sure because even fresh raw food these days might be spoiled due to wrong storage, delivery or harvesting issues. So we have our responsibility to decide how to eat and what to eat. I want here to share with you the imagination of how minerals and vitamins eaten from the piece of carrot in certain quantity will get to your body, will be digested and will be transformed to your cells, literally means to your body and soon they will become a part of your body by means of certain cells. This is why we say "we are what we eat". As you understand, all the rest, for example cellulose will go out as an absolutely unnecessary product. This is the difference between animal food and veg ones, all the unnecessary products will be absolutely excluded from our body and our digestive system will keep some of that cellulose inside only in cases of some digestive disorders, but in regular cases all food goes away. You may pay attention that we may visit restroom faster and more often after taking veg food comparing to animal ones. When we eat flesh, all unnecessary products are not easily removed from our body because of more complicated structure and we all know that necessary time for digestion of vegetables is around an hour or two and digestion time for meat may be easily around six hours. This time will be enough to poison a bit our body, portion by portion from inside, because unused products still remain in our digestive system and they start being spoiled inside, and all this leads to the dysfunction in our digestion ability, which may lead to losing lots of other elements from other food. The benefit is clear; we teach our body to be more clean and sensitive to consumption the useful elements and be able to take maximum available and stay clean. A skin condition may be an indication, when it is becoming more clear with the soft touch, full of live and natural colours. This is how we help our body to digest for us properly.

How can we follow consumption of proteins and have calories balanced? We have to understand the properties of food we take.

It is considerable to start with proteins as one of the necessary and fairly contradictious elements. I made table for myself and kindly share it with you, it can help you a lot or you can create your own one based on your habits, local food possibilities and other factors. This table does not guarantee the way you need and that it will work for you certainly, and again, I would like to show it as an example in which way you may follow your diet and be organized in healthy organic way.

Protein table.

Table of food properties for getting more protein per 100 grams (3.52oz) (information is based on dry raw products)

Table is given as an example and there is much more variety in food

Product	protein	Carbs	Fats	Calories
Seitan*	55g (1.94oz)	20.3g(0.71oz)	3.5g(0.12oz)	307 kcal
Yellow peas	20 g (0.70oz)	53.3g(1.88oz)	2.0g(0.07oz)	298 kcal
Lentils(mix color)	24 g (0.84oz)	42.7g(1.50oz)	1.5g(0.05oz)	284 kcal
White beans	21 g(0.74oz)	64.0g(2.25oz)	1.8g(0.06oz)	325 kcal
Chickpea	19 g(0.67oz)	61.0g(2.15oz)	6.0g(0.21oz)	364 kcal
Quinoa	14 g(0.49oz)	57.2g(2.01oz)	6.1g(0.21oz)	368 kcal
White rice	6.4g(0.22oz)	78.9g(2.78oz)	0.7g(0.02oz)	344 kcal
Red beans	8.4g(0.29oz)	13.7g(0.48oz)	0.3g(0.01oz)	93 kcal
Black beans	8.9g(0.31oz)	23.7g(0.83oz)	0.5g(0.01oz)	132 kcal
Cheese Tofu	8.1g(0.28oz)	0.6 g(0.02oz)	4.2g(0.14oz)	73 kcal
Green peas	5.0g(0.17oz)	13.8g(0.48oz)	0.2g(0.01oz)	73 kcal

* Seitan should be taken only in case if there is no allergy to gluten

Low calories products

Product	protein	Carbs	Fats	Calories
Blackeyed peas	2.8g(0.09oz)	8.4g(0.29oz)	0.4g(0.01oz)	47 kcal
Broccoli	3.0g(0.10oz)	5.2g(0.18oz)	0.4g(0.01oz)	28 kcal
Asparagus	1.9g(0.06oz)	3.1g(0.10oz)	0.1g(0.01oz)	20 kcal
Banana	1.5g(0.05oz)	1.5g(0.05oz)	0.2g(0.01oz)	95 kcal
Dried apricot	5.2g(0.18oz)	51.0g(1.79oz)	0.3g(0.01oz)	215 kcal

I divided this table into two parts: products with high volume of calories and proteins as well (the first part), and products with less calories (second part). From this information you may conclude how beneficial different types of food may be for you. Let me give you an example. An average person daily requirement of calories is somewhere between 1500 to 2000 kcal (this number depends on the gender, age, lifestyle). Many different factors should be considered separately. Let us take the minimum average level of 1500 kcal per person a day divided into average 3 meals per day. In this case we have 1500 / 3 makes 500 kcal per one meal. We have to respect different proportions for breakfast, lunch and dinner. Most of the specialists claim that breakfast should be the biggest part and be around 40% (some of them say that even 50% of the whole daily portion). If we refer to 40% from 1500 kcal it means we should take around 600 kcal for breakfast, for lunch we have around 500 kcal and around 400 we have for dinner. Again, this is quite individual aspect and we have to consider our own way of meal plan according to other many factors. So, from this example, I know that I have to take around 600 kcal in the morning for my breakfast, and I have a product list that I usually eat and I have to choose. Since we know that in order to reduce weight, we need to decrease calories and in order to gain weight we have to increase calories. If I want to increase calories, I choose high calories food, and usually, if I want to increase muscles, I need to pay attention to high volume of proteins in food. The leader in proteins, carbs and fats combination is seitan. So, consumption of 100g (3.52oz) of this product will give you 55g (1.94oz) of proteins and only 20g (0.70oz) of carbs. Of course, we need to pay attention that there is a big amount of calories, but 55g (1.94oz) of proteins will cost you 307 kcal. Since we take 600 kcal per breakfast, we can add another 100g (3.52oz) of additional product to our seitan, for instance lentils or quinoa where you can get another 20g (0.70oz) of proteins, 50g (1.76oz) of carbs and another 300 kcal. All the numbers are approximate and depend on the way of cooking and some additional elements in meal like oils or vegetables. So, we get 200g (7.05oz) of meal and 600 kcal where we get around 70g (2.46oz) of proteins and around 70g (2.46oz) of carbs and low fat (in general it will be around 10g (0.35oz)). Many diet specialists claim that the best proportion is 30g (1.05oz) of proteins, 50g (1.76oz) of carbs and 20g (0.70oz) of fats for any 100g (3.52oz). It means that meal containing seitan will have proportion of 35g (1.23oz) of proteins, 35 (1.23oz) of carbs and 10 (0.35oz) of fats, and we may consider this type of meal as low carb and low fat meal with lots of proteins. I think this type of meal is good for gaining muscles, but not for weight loss. When we speak about weight loss, it is not only about calories and fats, proteins are easily transformed to fats like carbs, if they are not used properly and energy is not spent or there is some metabolic disorder. Many factors may be involved and we have to consider them all. But we have to start with something. Many people never think about how they eat and what they eat and then, when they decide to move to vegetarian life they are lost in the woods of theories and completely lost in a knowledge of formation and transformation of our food. They just stop eating flesh, but what is next? First, what people come across with, when they stop eating flesh is a disproportion of elements. Usually, people go towards carbs and the reason for that is that they want a substantial food same way as they want something delicious. Sugar based goods come to help. This is not the way to do, and this is what happened to me, when I stopped eating flesh and I did not even feel that there was a problem with this and I ate a lot of carbs, especially in potatoes or cereals and grains. Then, I needed to increase my portions, because I wanted to fill full, and I needed my meals to be substantial. I didn't even notice how I gained another 20 kilo (44 pounds) to my body so fast and so easily. This process was so fast and easy and so complicated in reverse.

If you never watched what and how you eat, do it, especially when you change for vegetarian way of life. Besides this, you need to use energy as fast as you eat and physical activity may be a good friend.

Another example of food combination can be red beans and lentils and, if you do the same calculation from the above mentioned table, you will understand that from 200g (7.05oz) of food you will get around 300 kcal which is good for weight loss. Together with this, you will get fewer proteins and you will feel the food to be less substantial, and be ready for this, because you need to change your psychological state of mind to something else in order to forget about the food. One of the reasons, why you will feel less substantial will be lack of proteins (in case with lentils plus red beans, you will have around 30g (1.05oz) of proteins, which is not the worst result, but for some meat eaters might be difficult at the beginning)

If you are good with dairy products and you still eat them, you may also pay attention to the very big source of proteins in the following table below; it may give you an additional source of proteins which will make your food more substantial:

Dairy protein table

Table is given as an example and there is much more variety in food

Product	protein	Carbs	Fats	Calories
Gouda cheese	25g (0.88oz)	2.0g(0.07oz)	27g(0.95oz)	356 kcal
Mozzarella cheese	18g (0.63oz)	0.0g(0.00oz)	24g(0.84oz)	240 kcal
Camembert cheese	21g (0.74oz)	0.0g(0.00oz)	23g(0.81oz)	291 kcal

Carbohydrates.

This type of elements is the source of energy for us and this is why every product obviously contains it.

Carbohydrates table

Table of food properties for getting carbohydrates per 100 grams (information is based on dry raw products).

Product	protein	Carbs	Fats	Calories
Buckwheat	12g (1.94oz)	62.1g(2.19oz)	3.3g(0.12oz)	313 kcal
Oats	12g (1.94oz)	59.5g(2.09oz)	6.1g(0.21oz)	342 kcal
Wheat grains	11g (0.38oz)	59.5g(2.09oz)	2.2g(0.07oz)	342 kcal
Barley groats	10g (0.35oz)	71.7g(2.52oz)	1.3g(0.04oz)	324 kcal
Pearl barley	9g (0.31oz)	73.7g(2.59oz)	1.1g(0.03oz)	320 kcal
Corn grits	8g (0.28oz)	75.0g(2.64oz)	1.2g(0.04oz)	337 kcal

The information on carbohydrates is useful in case, if you really feel the deficit of carbs and mostly need to gain weight. These carbs also contain proteins which are always good for us in any way, because proteins contain amino acids and amino acids help us a lot. From another point, you cannot feed yourself only with some specific types of food, and you will need variety, so this information is useful for you to know what will happen, if you eat oats or buckwheat, for instance. Again, we speak all the time about calories as the fundamental issue in weight control and there is another recommendation stating that it is better to eat more carbs in the morning and less carbs in the evening in favour of protein. So it is normal to eat oats in the morning and get 60g (2.11oz) of carbs and 12g (0.42oz) of proteins, and if you eat 200g (7.05oz) of oats served with some berries and other fruits on your taste, you will finally get around 700 - 750 kcal, depending on serving type. This can be your normal size of your morning portion.

There is another point in carbs which goes to so-called fast and slow carbs. We are not going to study the complicated theory of different types in so detailed way, and go to glycemic index of each product. I will show you easier way to understand those different types. Everything as sweets, and not only sweets, also broad variety of cakes and chocolates can be considered as fast carbs as well. Some fruits are of high level as well. So, high glycemic index of food means that the food will be digested very fast and only some glucose will be taken for the energy consumption, all the rest will be saved as fat in our body. Slow carbs are the food with low glycemic index, which leads to slow digestion taking more carbs and glucose as well in favour of energy and not to save as fat for a longer period of time. Evolution made us do it for only one famous reason, back in time people used to eat very rarely with big intervals between meals and in order to survive; they had to save energy in a special form, transforming it into fat. After some time, we are able to have meals much more often and we eliminated huge intervals and changed our habits, but results of evolution are still in us. Speaking about slow carbs, we eat food in a manner to give our body a chance to use the carbs as postponed energy, and since we act during the day and we do something physically, we simply need the energy for all of this. When slow carbs are digested slowly, it means that we have more time to feel full and more energy in us for hours. There is a big difference between eating oats with berries and eating cakes. Oats will give us at least couple of hours of pure energy and it will not be stored into fat easily and cake with lots of sugar will give us 20-30 min of pure energy and all the rest will be stored in fats. In order to understand this, it is very simple to demonstrate, when we compare the same 200g (7.05oz) of oats, even served with fruits and honey and 200g (7.05oz) of cake. First, the quantity of calories in cake will be higher, depending on type of cake, of course, but still, let's accept that there is the same level of calories - 750 kcal. Oats will be using those 750 kcal for at least two hours and we will feel full during all this time, and if we walk during one hour, it means that we will burn around 300 kcal per hour, so you may be sure that approximately 100g (3.52oz) of oats will be used for energy to walk and not to store. Since oats are slow carbs we have another one hour to dance and burn another 100g (3.52oz) of oats, because we have two hours of our time to use carbs for energy. It is known as a glycemic window, in other words. It is the time given to burn calories in the most effective way. Not all energy will be used, depending on the activity type and hormones and other personal characteristics, but the idea is clear. Now, let's see an example with 750 kcal of cake. Our window will be only 30 minutes to burn all 750 kcal, if we don't burn them, all the rest goes to a fat store. Can you imagine, how fast should you run and how intensively you should do it right after eating cakes? I have doubts that some of us can do that. First, we don't have time to do so. So, during the time of 30 min we will burn only 150 kcal and all the rest (600 kcal) will be used to fat store after those half an hour. Of course, it is not so strict, and if we don't eat cake during the day after breakfast, we may have a chance to use those 600 kcal, because there will be no other food and the body will start using the strategic storage of fat to give energy to a body. Question is where it is using it from. The trick is that it is using it from the muscles, destructing them first and then it will use fat only at the second stage. This is our cunning evolution and nature that created it with an absolute logic and wisdom. So, a good excuse about eating cakes in the morning is only an excuse, because practically it does not matter so much due to the very short glycaemic period of time. Of course, the chance to use more energy in the morning is higher than in the evening, but still not so important. I feel indignation from many of you about this ascetic way of life and full denying of eating fast carbs. For sure, we should not deny, and on the contrary, I must admit that we eat those things, question lays in our habits and motivation. If we are motivated to have sound and healthy body meaning soul as well, we will eat them, but not quite often and everything will be under total control by us. We need to understand, even feel this that habits should control habits, but habits should not control us. How? One of the instruments can be 21 days to change habit and you may trust me and my experience saying that this is possible. You just need to have a goal and understand what you do. If you are a big sugar eater, find natural healthy food to substitute sugar based products and do 21 no sugar days, but eat something which will help you not to go crazy. If you have a habit to drink tea with sugar in the morning, use stevia herb instead, taste is almost the same, but sugar is zero. You may do some own experiments and find the best range of food for you to run those 21 days. At the end of 21 days, you may feel that you like the way you do, and you may feel like you don't want to go back. For sure, there is no promise that it will work for you at the first time and you will change so fast, it depends on how strong your habit is and your psychological deepness, but in most cases, it helps. If you feel no change, be honest to yourself and just don't give up and do it again after some time, you will obviously change. I always think that if other people are able to do something, I am personally able to do the same. This is why we share experience with people even though we are all different and the result definitely will come. This 21 days instrument is so powerful that it can give us a lot of help in our way of changing our habit to better things.

Fats.

Fats are absolutely necessary for us, especially in case of change to vegetarian life. We speak about different types of fats, and again the big volume of them are found in animal products, and if you are not going to eat meat, fish or eggs you may change to dairy products like cottage cheese or mozzarella or any other type of cheese, which contain specifically a lot of fats, useful fats or monounsaturated fats found in some vegetables, fruits, oils and nuts. I will pay attention to some very important sources of fats, which you may miss in case of being vegetarian.

If we stop eating fish, we start to lack Omega 3 and 6. One of the best sources of Omega is a chia seed. Another one can be natural hemp oil; the third one is a flax seed. All of them are almost on the same level of saturation. And again, since we take control over our calories, we need to know the price for getting useful fats. Here, I would like to pay attention from my own experience. There is no way to exclude fats from your meal, if you want to control weight, control calories and do not exclude fats. I mean, there is no sense to exclude fatty yogurt or milk or any type of cheese. There is a bigger possibility that you will get even more calories or sugar saturated goods, which can be worse for your body, even in case of less calories, if you take low fat products. You should remember also about speed of digestion and use of those calories and how fast those calories are. So, this is a big question and it is your own decision what to do, but I decided not to exclude fats from my meals.

So when, I eat oats in the morning, I add there chia seed or flax seeds, each day can be different. Those seeds are big in calories, but do not worry so much about calories, you will not eat more than 50 kcal, because volume for 100g (3.52oz) of seeds should be very big and it is rather hard to eat a lot of seeds, oils or nuts. Only in case, if you are real lover of beer and real nutcracker, yes, you have to pay attention to what you eat and how many, because eating nuts without control may bring you to a huge amount of calories.

So, let's see the table in order to know how to control our calories from general tasty sources of fats.

Fats table

Product	protein	Carbs	Fats	Calories
Olive oil	0g (0.00oz)	0.0g(2.09oz)	99g(3.52oz)	898 kcal
Flax oil	0g (0.00oz)	0.0g(2.09oz)	99g(3.52oz)	898 kcal
Hazelnut	15g (0.52oz)	9.9g(0.34oz)	66g(2.32oz)	704 kcal
Pecan walnut	9g (0.31oz)	4.3g(0.15oz)	72g(2.53oz)	691 kcal
Walnut	15g (0.52oz)	7.0g(0.24oz)	65g(2.20oz)	654 kcal
Peanuts	26g (0.91oz)	9.9g(0.34oz)	45g(0.58oz)	622 kcal
Pistachios	20g (0.70oz)	7.0g(0.24oz)	50g(1.76oz)	556 kcal
Flax seeds	18g (0.63oz)	28.9g(1.01oz)	42g(1.48oz)	534 kcal
Chia seeds	16g (0.56oz)	30g(1.05oz)	42.1g(1.48oz)	512 kcal
Sweet almond	18g (0.63oz)	16.2g(0.57oz)	57g(2.01oz)	645 kcal
Cashew	18g (0.63oz)	22.5g(0.79oz)	48g(1.69oz)	600 kcal
Macadamia Nut	8g (0.28oz)	5.2g(0.18oz)	75g(2.64oz)	718 kcal
Coconut	3g (0.10oz)	6.2g(0.21oz)	33g(1.16oz)	354 kcal
Chestnut	3g (0.10oz)	3g(0.10oz)	30.6g(1.07oz)	354 kcal

I would like to come back to importance of fats in nuts and Omega, specifically Omega 3. The fact is that we are receiving Omega 6 much easier than Omega 3 and nuts and oils are giving us very good proportion of Omega 3 and 6 in the way that we are going to receive normal part of them easily. When we eat red fish and receive Omega, mostly we get Omega 6 and much less Omega 3. So in order to balance, we need some veggies Omega and nuts and oils are real helpers. Why is this acid so important for us? This question is in the area of our blood system. Omega 3 acids help our blood vessels to be in normal condition. So called "bad cholesterol" is eliminated by effective work of Omega 3. Another example is Lauric acid, which is found in coconut. This outstanding acid transforms saturated fats into monounsaturated and this is clear usefulness. Besides the Lauric acid, it is a good antimicrobial remedy. It is another big benefit to be vegetarian or even vegan when we stop eating animal fats which are in most cases saturated ones leading to a bad cholesterol level.

Besides acids, the nuts, the seeds and the oils are enriched with vitamins of different types, the coconut has vitamin A, B1, B9, B12 and many others, the walnut is enriched with A, B1, B2, B5, B6, B9, C, E, and K plus, it is full of minerals like potassium, calcium, magnesium, zinc, selenium, copper and manganese, iron, phosphorus and sodium. The flax oil is enriched with polyunsaturated Omega 3, Omega 6 and Omega 9 acids. It is also very important to mention that any heating of flax oil is prohibited, because this oil will produce carcinogens when heated or even exposed to the sun. This is why this oil should be stored properly with no sunlight exposure. It should be stored in dry dark and even better cold place, so the fridge will be enough, and if the bottle is open, it should not be stored longer than three months after opening. Please, consider this as a very important message in order not to transform useful oil to rubbish. Normally, no oil should be heated, because of the same properties, only special oils which are intended for frying or other heating can be used in any heating manipulations.

We are coming to the last chapter of the book, and it is related to the heating. I hope the information which was given above can be useful for you and you will understand the idea of calories control. I am not touching vegetables, because it is clear that we need them, we eat them and they do not have so many calories comparing to the products listed above. My idea is to show you the products that you will be able to use in order to substitute flesh and get the most efficient and substantial elements for yourself. So, now you can understand how much this or that meal can bring for you, and what it will bring depending on your goals. Please, consider also that the information given in the table cannot be used as an exact recommendation. Many things depend on food preparation, meal type, combination of meals and even such factors like temperature.

Fire.

This is the last chapter of this book, touching very interesting aspect of our life. This aspect is a use of fire. People used fire from the ancient times, fire heated people, fire destroyed everything around and fire terminated harmful bacteria in the food. People found that eating food cooked on fire is more delicious and safer. This is an absolute true! This is true to any animal products, specifically when we eat the flesh. But this is absolutely not true for eating veggie food. It is simply enough to splash it with pure water in the most cases. I am not speaking today about the cases when we have food full of chemicals and we need to boil it sometimes, because pure water is not enough, but in regular and natural cases, it is enough and absolutely ok to use only water.

Many people following the idea of raw food today. This idea is preceded in the most cases by vegetarianism, when people stop to feel the importance of cooking food on fire and keep all the vitamins and elements in a raw food. Of course, there are many ways of eating raw food today and people created the ways to eat raw flesh previously made with all possible preservatives and bacteria eliminators, but this is an extraordinary topic which is not the part of our book.

There are two theories existing about raw food importance. One is natural and biological and another one is biological and esoteric. So, natural idea goes to keeping preserved all possible elements in food before we put it into our mouth. And, this is true, since my childhood I heard that the best fruit is the one ripped from the tree right away before eating in the garden. After several days of being in the basket, taken from the market and stored at home it loses around fifty percent of all useful minerals and vitamins, and if we cook this fruit it will lose almost everything. We usually do not boil or fry fruits so commonly, but vegetables we do and quite often we do. In every cuisine of almost any nation you may find different recipes of cooking vegetables. Raw eaters still believe that the best way to eat such veggie food is to get it fresh and not cooked.

Another question comes to cereals and different types of porridge. First of all there are different ways to cook such food today and technologies are helping us a lot, so we can dry food or use a food steamer. In case with potato or rice, most of us are unable to eat it raw, and this is even not delicious, so drier or steamer can be the best solution.

The followers of esoteric way, believe that fire is transforming energy in the food structure, because it eliminates and transform the energy in the food as well, it changes its structure and destroys all the useful elements in food. Fire is used in many practices and used in meditations in order to eliminate bad emotions or feelings, since ancient times people knew it and used it alongside with heating or cooking. Spiritual use of fire can be found in every culture and this is not a big secret. I personally believe into both versions, and as I mentioned already in this book, everything is energy and every element is an energy and we are all the same energy, the difference is only its physical aspect, which is depicted in food, things around, animals, trees whatever else. You know that strong fire transforms sand into glass, so it works with the same energy and simply transforms it. Energy is not eliminated, but it is transformed into different aspect and changes its physical properties as a result. Here, we may think of this idea again and we can agree that nature gives us a tomato or a cucumber full of different properties useful for our bodies and they are formed in a certain way for us. So, there is no sense to change those properties by fire and do it instead of nature. Since every element brings us the element of energy, it is like a copy to a physical form of the thing, and since we are not able to see it, we often deny its existence seeing only physical form. Do you remember that we are what we eat? How? It is simple. Minerals are becoming a part of our body helping us in our development and the energy of the minerals becomes a part of our energy body. It is invisible, but it does not mean that it does not exist, and personally for me after many practices, I have no doubts in its existence.

In conclusion, if you have a possibility and your physical condition allows you to have a raw food; you'd better prefer the raw food to the cooked one.

I hope my small experience will help you with your starting, progression and it will make things more clear and conscious for you.

In my next series, I will do my best to share my cooking experience with you, providing the most delicious and easy way, so follow me and I wish you a good luck, a lot of wisdom, light and positiveness.

Many people in the world practicing meditations, yoga or any spiritual practices that make a huge change to entire Planet by means of changing own mind, surrounding and attitude.

THANK YOU!